The Biography of
Florence Nightingale

The Biography of Florence Nightingale

by Lytton Strachey
With an Introduction by Anita S. Kessler, R.N., M.S.N., M.Ed.

©2008 Wilder Publications

A & D Publishing
PO Box 3005
Radford VA 24143-3005
www.wilderpublications.com

ISBN 10: 1-60459-207-9
ISBN 13: 978-1-60459-207-8

First Edition

Introduction

As a nurse, I had my own ideas of what Florence Nightingale must have been like as a nurse and as a person. Strachey's biography both confirmed and challenged most of these beliefs. I was surprised and shocked to learn some of the information I read about Miss Nightingale.

Have you wondered how as a woman, she accomplished so much in her lifetime over a century ago? What have women, and nurses especially, had to do in the last sixty years to enjoy the independence and recognition of nursing as a true profession? Imagine how much harder that would have been in the mid-nineteenth century!

Yes, she was a healer, a comforter, and a nurturer. But like all of us, she had a dark side. That was a part of her life I personally found fascinating in this biography. What was in her "shadow" as Carl Jung would have asked? Was she assertive or overly aggressive? Did she open up opportunities with important people to further her cause or did she "use them"? Just how charismatic was she? She was spiritual, but how did she really feel about Christianityl? What was her relationship with God as she knew him? Why did she not have a woman as her assistant/secretary?

This is not an autobiography so how did Lytton Strachey get his information? He used the writings from her personal journals, the writings of the men she influenced and interviews with those that knew her. His historical presentation of the Crimean war, England, and socio-cultural views is very accurate and correlates with what I personally have read before. But his knowledge and insights about Florence Nightingale are more thorough and different than I have been taught.

If you are a nurse, or are becoming a nurse, you should read this biography. It caused me to question whether I would agree or disagree with the author's analyses. In the end, I believe I am more in awe, more proud of what Ms. Nightingale accomplished than I was before I read the biography. I also have a greater understanding of the passion, drive and love of work she exhibited. Yes, she had a "dark" side; don't we all? Her mystique, her charisma were in part because she could use this darkness to get what she wanted. Seldom, did anyone really know her. They were drawn to her. They had to be with her. They admired her. At least one man literally worked himself to death for her. There is no doubt she was a force with which one had to attend. Denial of her passion and abilities generally led only to personal devastation in one way or another!

She is legend. She is real, faults and all. Don't you want to understand her better? This book will help you to do that. Form your own conclusions about our leader of modern day nursing. It will give you a deeper appreciation of what we have today in the profession of nursing.

Anita S. Kessler, R.N., M.S.N., M.Ed. Nurse Educator

EVERY one knows the popular conception of Florence Nightingale. The saintly, self-sacrificing woman, the delicate maiden of high degree who threw aside the pleasures of a life of ease to succour the afflicted; the Lady with the Lamp, gliding through the horrors of the hospital at Scutari, and consecrating with the radiance of her goodness the dying soldier's couch. The vision is familiar to all—but the truth was different. The Miss Nightingale of fact was not as facile as fancy painted her. She worked in another fashion and towards another end; she moved under the stress of an impetus which finds no place in the popular imagination. A Demon possessed her. Now demons, whatever else they may be, are full of interest. And so it happens that in the real Miss Nightingale there was more that was interesting than in the legendary one; there was also less that was agreeable.

Her family was extremely well-to-do, and connected by marriage with a spreading circle of other well-to-do families. There was a large country house in Derbyshire; there was another in the New Forest; there were Mayfair rooms for the London season and all its finest parties; there were tours on the Continent with even more than the usual number of Italian operas and of glimpses at the celebrities of Paris. Brought up among such advantages, it was only natural to suppose that Florence would show a proper appreciation of them by doing her duty in that state of life unto which it had pleased God to call her—in other words, by marrying, after a fitting number of dances and dinner-parties, an eligible gentleman, and living happily ever afterwards. Her sister, her cousins, all the young ladies of her acquaintance, were either getting ready to do this or had already done it.

It was inconceivable that Florence should dream of anything else; yet dream she did. Ah! To do her duty in that state of life unto which it had pleased God to call her! Assuredly, she would not be behindhand in doing her duty; but unto what state of life HAD it pleased God to call her? That was the question. God's calls are many, and they are strange. Unto what state of life had it pleased Him to call Charlotte Corday, or Elizabeth of Hungary? What was that secret voice in her ear, if it was not a call? Why had she felt, from her earliest years, those mysterious promptings towards... she hardly knew what, but certainly towards something very different from anything around her? Why, as a child in the nursery, when her sister had shown a healthy pleasure in tearing her dolls to pieces, had SHE shown an almost morbid one in sewing them up again? Why was she driven now to minister to the poor in their cottages, to watch by sick-beds, to put her dog's wounded paw into elaborate splints as if it was a human being? Why was her head filled with queer imaginations of the country house at Embley turned, by some enchantment, into a hospital, with herself as matron moving about among the beds? Why was even her vision of heaven itself filled with suffering patients to whom she was being useful? So she dreamed and wondered, and, taking out her diary, she poured into it the agitations of her soul. And then the bell rang, and it was time to go and dress for dinner.

As the years passed, a restlessness began to grow upon her. She was unhappy, and at last she knew it. Mrs. Nightingale, too, began to notice that there was something wrong. It was very odd— what could be

the matter with dear Flo? Mr. Nightingale suggested
that a husband might be advisable; but the curious
thing was that she seemed to take no interest in
husbands. And with her attractions, and her
accomplishments, too! There was nothing in the
world to prevent her making a really brilliant
match. But no! She would think of nothing but how
to satisfy that singular craving of hers to be DOING
something. As if there was not plenty to do in any
case, in the ordinary way, at home. There was the
china to look after, and there was her father to be
read to after dinner. Mrs. Nightingale could not
understand it; and then one day her perplexity was
changed to consternation and alarm. Florence
announced an extreme desire to go to Salisbury
Hospital for several months as a nurse; and she
confessed to some visionary plan of eventually
setting up in a house of her own in a neighbouring
village, and there founding 'something like a
Protestant Sisterhood, without vows, for women of
educated feelings'. The whole scheme was
summarily brushed aside as preposterous; and Mrs.
Nightingale, after the first shock of terror, was able
to settle down again more or less comfortably to her
embroidery. But Florence, who was now twenty-five
and felt that the dream of her life had been
shattered, came near to desperation.

And, indeed, the difficulties in her path were
great. For not only was it an almost unimaginable
thing in those days for a woman of means to make
her own way in the world and to live in
independence, but the particular profession for
which Florence was clearly marked out both by her
instincts and her capacities was at that time a
peculiarly disreputable one. A 'nurse' meant then a
coarse old woman, always ignorant, usually dirty,

often brutal, a Mrs. Gamp, in bunched-up sordid garments, tippling at the brandy bottle or indulging in worse irregularities. The nurses in the hospitals were especially notorious for immoral conduct; sobriety was almost unknown among them; and they could hardly be trusted to carry out the simplest medical duties.

Certainly, things HAVE changed since those days; and that they have changed is due, far more than to any other human being, to Miss Nightingale herself. It is not to be wondered at that her parents should have shuddered at the notion of their daughter devoting her life to such an occupation. 'It was as if,' she herself said afterwards, 'I had wanted to be a kitchen-maid.' Yet the want, absurd and impracticable as it was, not only remained fixed immovably in her heart, but grew in intensity day by day. Her wretchedness deepened into a morbid melancholy. Everything about her was vile, and she herself, it was clear, to have deserved such misery, was even viler than her surroundings. Yes, she had sinned—'standing before God's judgment seat'. 'No one,' she declared, 'has so grieved the Holy Spirit'; of that she was quite certain. It was in vain that she prayed to be delivered from vanity and hypocrisy, and she could not bear to smile or to be gay, 'because she hated God to hear her laugh, as if she had not repented of her sin'.

A weaker spirit would have been overwhelmed by the load of such distresses— would have yielded or snapped. But this extraordinary young woman held firm, and fought her way to victory. With an amazing persistency, during the eight years that followed her rebuff over Salisbury Hospital, she struggled and worked and planned. While superficially she was carrying on the life of a brilliant girl in high society, while internally she was a prey to the tortures of regret and of remorse, she yet possessed the energy to collect the knowledge and to undergo the experience which alone could enable her to do what she had determined she would do in the end. In secret she devoured the reports of medical commissions, the pamphlets of sanitary authorities, the histories of hospitals and homes. She spent the intervals of the London season in ragged schools and workhouses. When she went abroad with her family, she used her spare time so well that there was hardly a great hospital in Europe with which she was not acquainted; hardly a great city whose shims she had not passed through. She managed to spend some days in a convent school in Rome, and some weeks as a 'Soeur de Charite' in Paris. Then, while her mother and sister were taking the waters at Carlsbad, she succeeded in slipping off to a nursing institution at Kaiserswerth, where she remained for more than three months. This was the critical event of her life. The experience which she gained as a nurse at Kaiserswerth formed the foundation of all her future action and finally fixed her in her career.

But one other trial awaited her. The allurements of the world she had brushed aside with disdain and loathing; she had resisted the subtler temptation which, in her weariness, had sometimes come upon her, of devoting her baffled energies to art or literature; the last ordeal appeared in the shape of a desirable young man. Hitherto, her lovers had been nothing to her but an added burden and a mockery; but now— for a moment— she wavered. A new feeling swept over her—a feeling which she had never known before— which she was never to know again. The most powerful and the profoundest of all the instincts of humanity laid claim upon her. But it rose before her, that instinct, arrayed—how could it be otherwise?— in the inevitable habiliments of a Victorian marriage; and she had the strength to stamp it underfoot. 'I have an intellectual nature which requires satisfaction,' she noted, 'and that would find it in him. I have a passionate nature which requires satisfaction, and that would find it in him. I have a moral, an active nature which requires satisfaction, and that would not find it in his life. Sometimes I think that I will satisfy my passionate nature at all events. ...'

But no, she knew in her heart that it could not be. 'To be nailed to a continuation and exaggeration of my present life ... to put it out of my power ever to be able to seize the chance of forming for myself a true and rich life'—that would be a suicide. She made her choice, and refused what was at least a certain happiness for a visionary good which might never come to her at all. And so she returned to her old life of waiting and bitterness. 'The thoughts and feelings that I have now,' she wrote, 'I can remember since I was six years old. A profession, a trade, a necessary occupation, something to fill and employ all my faculties, I have always felt essential to me, I have always longed for. The first thought I can remember, and the last, was nursing work; and in the absence of this, education work, but more the education of the bad than of the young... Everything has been tried— foreign travel, kind friends, everything. My God! What is to become of me?' A desirable young man? Dust and ashes! What was there desirable in such a thing as that? 'In my thirty-first year,' she noted in her diary, 'I see nothing desirable but death.'

Three more years passed, and then at last the

pressure of time told; her family seemed to realise that she was old enough and strong enough to have her way; and she became the superintendent of a charitable nursing home in Harley Street. She had gained her independence, though it was in a meagre sphere enough; and her mother was still not quite resigned: surely Florence might at least spend the summer in the country. At times, indeed, among her intimates, Mrs. Nightingale almost wept. 'We are ducks,' she said with tears in her eyes, 'who have hatched a wild swan.' But the poor lady was wrong; it was not a swan that they had hatched, it was an eagle.

II

Miss NIGHTINGALE had been a year in her nursing-home in Harley Street, when Fate knocked at the door. The Crimean War broke out; the battle of the Alma was fought; and the terrible condition of our military hospitals at Scutari began to be known in England. It sometimes happens that the plans of Providence are a little difficult to follow, but on this occasion all was plain; there was a perfect coordination of events. For years Miss Nightingale had been getting ready; at last she was prepared— experienced, free, mature, yet still young (she was thirty-four)— desirous to serve, accustomed to command: at that precise moment the desperate need of a great nation came, and she was there to satisfy it. If the war had fallen a few years earlier, she would have lacked the knowledge, perhaps even the power, for such a work; a few years later and she would, no doubt, have been fixed in the routine of some absorbing task, and moreover, she would have been growing old.

Nor was it only the coincidence of time that was remarkable. It so fell out that Sidney Herbert was at the War Office and in the Cabinet; and Sidney Herbert was an intimate friend of Miss Nightingale's, convinced, from personal experience in charitable work, of her supreme capacity. After such premises, it seems hardly more than a matter of course that her letter, in which she offered her services for the East, and Sidney Herbert's letter, in which he asked for them, should actually have crossed in the post. Thus it all happened, without a hitch. The appointment was made and even Mrs. Nightingale, overawed by the magnitude of the venture, could only approve. A pair of faithful friends offered themselves as personal attendants; thirty-eight nurses were collected; and within a week of the crossing of the letters Miss Nightingale, amid a great burst of popular enthusiasm, left for Constantinople.

Among the numerous letters which she received on her departure was one from Dr. Manning, who at that time was working in comparative obscurity as a Catholic priest in Bayswater. 'God will keep you,' he wrote, 'and my prayer for you will be that your one object of worship, Pattern of Imitation, and source of consolation and strength, may be the Sacred Heart of our Divine Lord.'

To what extent Dr. Manning's prayer was answered must remain a matter of doubt; but this much is certain: that if ever a prayer was needed, it was needed then for Florence Nightingale. For dark as had been the picture of the state of affairs at Scutari, revealed to the English public in the dispatches of "The Times Correspondent", and in a multitude of private letters, yet the reality turned out to be darker still. What had occurred was, in brief, the complete breakdown of our medical arrangements at the seat of war. The origins of this awful failure were complex and manifold; they stretched back through long years of peace and carelessness in England; they could be traced through endless ramifications of administrative incapacity— from the inherent faults of confused systems, to the petty bunglings of minor officials, from the inevitable ignorance of Cabinet Ministers, to the fatal exactitudes of narrow routine.

In the inquiries which followed, it was clearly shown that the evil was in reality that worst of all evils— one which has been caused by nothing in particular and for which no one in particular is to blame. The whole organisation of the war machine was incompetent and out of date. The old Duke had sat for a generation at the Horse Guards repressing innovations with an iron hand. There was an extraordinary overlapping of authorities and an almost incredible shifting of responsibilities to and fro. As for such a notion as the creation and the maintenance of a really adequate medical service for the army— in that atmosphere of aged chaos, how could it have entered anybody's head? Before the war, the easygoing officials at Westminster were naturally persuaded that all was well— or at least as well as could be expected; when someone, for instance, actually had the temerity to suggest the formation of a corps of Army nurses, he was at once laughed out of court. When the war had begun, the gallant British officers in control of affairs had other things to think about than the petty details of medical organisation. Who had bothered with such trifles in the Peninsula? And surely, on that occasion, we had done pretty well. Thus, the most obvious precautions were neglected, and the most necessary preparations were put off from day to day. The principal medical officer of the Army, Dr. Hall, was summoned from India at a moment's notice, and was unable to visit England before taking up his duties at the front. And it was not until after the battle of the Alma, when we had been at war for many months, that we acquired hospital accommodations at Scutari for more than a thousand men. Errors, follies, and vices on the part of individuals there doubtless were; but, in the general reckoning, they were of small account— insignificant symptoms of the deep disease of the body politic— to the enormous calamity of administrative collapse.

Miss Nightingale arrived at Scutari— a suburb of Constantinople, on the Asiatic side of the Bosphorus— on November 4th, 1854; it was ten days after the battle of Balaclava, and the day before the battle of Inkerman. The organisation of the hospitals, which had already given way under the stress of the battle of the Alma, was now to be subjected to the further pressure which these two desperate and bloody engagements implied. Great detachments of wounded were already beginning to pour in. The men, after receiving such summary treatment as could be given them at the smaller hospitals in the Crimea itself, were forthwith shipped in batches of 200 across the Black Sea to Scutari. This voyage was in normal times one of four days and a half; but the times were no longer normal, and now the transit often lasted for a fortnight or three weeks. It received, not without reason, the name of the 'middle passage'. Between, and sometimes on the decks, the wounded, the sick, and the dying were crowded— men who had just undergone the amputation of limbs, men in the clutches of fever or of frostbite, men in the last stages of dysentry and cholera— without beds, sometimes without blankets, often hardly clothed. The one or two surgeons on board did what they could; but medical stores were lacking, and the only form of nursing available was that provided by a handful of invalid soldiers who were usually themselves prostrate by the end of the voyage. There was no other food beside the ordinary salt rations of ship diet; and even the water was sometimes so stored that it was out of reach of the weak. For many months, the average of deaths during these voyages was seventy-four in 1,000; the corpses were shot out into the waters; and who shall say that they were the most unfortunate? At Scutari, the landing-stage, constructed with all the perverseness of Oriental ingenuity, could only be approached with great difficulty, and, in rough weather, not at all. When it was reached, what remained of the men in the ships had first to be disembarked, and then conveyed up a steep slope of a quarter of a mile to the nearest of the hospitals. The most serious cases might be put upon stretchers— for there were far too few for all; the rest were carried or dragged up the hill by such convalescent soldiers as could be got together, who were not too obviously infirm for the work. At last the journey was accomplished; slowly, one by one, living or dying, the wounded were carried up into the hospital. And in the hospital what did they find?

Lasciate ogni speranza, voi ch'entrate: the delusive doors bore no such inscription; and yet behind them Hell yawned. Want, neglect, confusion, misery— in every shape and in every degree of intensity— filled the endless corridors and the vast apartments of the gigantic barrack-house, which, without forethought or preparation, had been hurriedly set aside as the chief shelter for the victims of the war. The very building itself was radically defective. Huge sewers underlay it, and cesspools loaded with filth wafted their poison into the upper rooms. The floors were in so rotten a condition that many of them could not be scrubbed; the walls were thick with dirt; incredible multitudes of vermin swarmed everywhere. And, enormous as the building was, it was yet too small. It contained four miles of beds, crushed together so close that there was but just room to pass between them. Under such conditions, the most elaborate system of ventilation might well have been at fault; but here there was no ventilation. The stench was indescribable. 'I have been well acquainted,' said Miss Nightingale, 'with the dwellings of the worst parts of most of the great cities in Europe, but have never been in any atmosphere which I could compare with that of the Barrack Hospital at night.' The structural defects were equalled by the deficiencies in the commonest objects of hospital use. There were not enough bedsteads; the sheets were of canvas, and so coarse that the wounded men recoiled from them, begging to be left in their blankets; there was no bedroom furniture of any kind, and empty beer bottles were used for candlesticks. There were no basins, no towels, no soap, no brooms, no mops, no trays, no plates; there were neither slippers nor scissors, neither shoe-brushes nor blacking; there were no knives or forks or spoons. The supply of fuel was constantly deficient. The cooking arrangements were preposterously inadequate, and the laundry was a farce. As for purely medical materials, the tale was no better. Stretchers, splints, bandages—all were lacking; and so were the most ordinary drugs.

To replace such wants, to struggle against such

difficulties, there was a handful of men
overburdened by the strain of ceaseless work, bound
down by the traditions of official routine, and
enfeebled either by old age or inexperience or sheer
incompetence. They had proved utterly unequal to
their task. The principal doctor was lost in the
imbecilities of a senile optimism. The wretched
official whose business it was to provide for the
wants of the hospital was tied fast hand and foot by
red tape. A few of the younger doctors struggled
valiantly, but what could they do? Unprepared,
disorganised, with such help only as they could find
among the miserable band of convalescent soldiers
drafted off to tend their sick comrades, they were
faced with disease, mutilation, and death in all their
most appalling forms, crowded multitudinously
about them in an ever-increasing mass. They were
like men in a shipwreck, fighting, not for safety, but
for the next moment's bare existence— to gain, by
yet another frenzied effort, some brief respite from
the waters of destruction.

In these surroundings, those who had been long
inured to scenes of human suffering—surgeons with
a world-wide knowledge of agonies, soldiers familiar
with fields of carnage, missionaries with
remembrances of famine and of plague— yet found
a depth of horror which they had never known
before. There were moments, there were places, in
the Barrack Hospital at Scutari, where the strongest
hand was struck with trembling, and the boldest eye
would turn away its gaze.

Miss Nightingale came, and she, at any rate, in
that inferno, did not abandon hope. For one thing,
she brought material succour. Before she left London
she had consulted Dr. Andrew Smith, the head of
the Army Medical Board, as to whether it would be

useful to take out stores of any kind to Scutari; and Dr. Andrew Smith had told her that 'nothing was needed'. Even Sidney Herbert had given her similar assurances; possibly, owing to an oversight, there might have been some delay in the delivery of the medical stores, which, he said, had been sent out from England 'in profusion', but 'four days would have remedied this'. She preferred to trust her own instincts, and at Marseilles purchased a large quantity of miscellaneous provisions, which were of the utmost use at Scutari. She came, too, amply provided with money— in all, during her stay in the East, about £7,000 reached her from private sources; and, in addition, she was able to avail herself of another valuable means of help.

At the same time as herself, Mr. Macdonald, of The Times, had arrived at Scutari, charged with the duty of administering the large sums of money collected through the agency of that newspaper in aid of the sick and wounded; and Mr. Macdonald had the sense to see that the best use he could make of The Times Fund was to put it at the disposal of Miss Nightingale. 'I cannot conceive,' wrote an eye-witness, 'as I now calmly look back on the first three weeks after the arrival of the wounded from Inkerman, how it could have been possible to have avoided a state of things too disastrous to contemplate, had not Miss Nightingale been there, with the means placed at her disposal by Mr. Macdonald.' But the official view was different. What! Was the public service to admit, by accepting outside charity, that it was unable to discharge its own duties without the assistance of private and irregular benevolence? Never! And accordingly when Lord Stratford de Redcliffe, our ambassador at Constantinople, was asked by Mr. Macdonald to indicate how The Times Fund could best be employed, he answered that there was indeed one object to which it might very well be devoted— the building of an English Protestant Church at Pera.

Mr. Macdonald did not waste further time with Lord Stratford, and immediately joined forces with Miss Nightingale. But, with such a frame of mind in the highest quarters, it is easy to imagine the kind of disgust and alarm with which the sudden intrusion of a band of amateurs and females must have filled the minds of the ordinary officer and the ordinary military surgeon. They could not understand it— what had women to do with war? Honest Colonels relieved their spleen by the cracking of heavy jokes about 'the Bird'; while poor Dr. Hall, a rough terrier of a man, who had worried his way to the top of his profession, was struck speechless with astonishment, and at last observed that Miss Nightingale's appointment was extremely droll.

Her position was, indeed, an official one, but it was hardly the easier for that. In the hospitals it was her duty to provide the services of herself and her nurses when they were asked for by the doctors, and not until then. At first some of the surgeons would have nothing to say to her, and, though she was welcomed by others, the majority were hostile and suspicious. But gradually she gained ground. Her good will could not be denied, and her capacity could not be disregarded. With consummate tact, with all the gentleness of supreme strength, she managed at last to impose her personality upon the susceptible, overwrought, discouraged, and helpless group of men in authority who surrounded her. She stood firm; she was a rock in the angry ocean; with her alone was safety, comfort, life. And so it was that hope dawned at Scutari. The reign of chaos and old night began to dwindle; order came upon the scene, and common sense, and forethought, and decision, radiating out from the little room off the great gallery in the Barrack Hospital where, day and night, the Lady Superintendent was at her task. Progress might be slow, but it was sure.

The first sign of a great change came with the appearance of some of those necessary objects with which the hospitals had been unprovided for months. The sick men began to enjoy the use of towels and soap, knives and forks, combs and tooth-brushes. Dr. Hall might snort when he heard of it, asking, with a growl, what a soldier wanted with a tooth-brush; but the good work went on. Eventually the whole business of purveying to the hospitals was, in effect, carried out by Miss Nightingale. She alone, it seemed. whatever the contingency, knew where to lay her hands on what was wanted; she alone could dispense her stores with readiness; above

all, she alone possessed the art of circumventing the pernicious influences of official etiquette. This was her greatest enemy, and sometimes even she was baffled by it. On one occasion 27,000 shirts, sent out at her instance by the Home Government, arrived, were landed, and were only waiting to be unpacked. But the official 'Purveyor' intervened; 'he could not unpack them,' he said, 'with out a Board.' Miss Nightingale pleaded in vain; the sick and wounded lay half-naked shivering for want of clothing; and three weeks elapsed before the Board released the shirts. A little later, however, on a similar occasion, Miss Nightingale felt that she could assert her own authority. She ordered a Government consignment to be forcibly opened while the miserable 'Purveyor' stood by, wringing his hands in departmental agony.

Vast quantities of valuable stores sent from England lay, she found, engulfed in the bottomless abyss of the Turkish Customs House. Other ship-loads, buried beneath munitions of war destined for Balaclava, passed Scutari without a sign, and thus hospital materials were sometimes carried to and fro three times over the Black Sea, before they reached their destination. The whole system was clearly at fault, and Miss Nightingale suggested to the home authorities that a Government Store House should be instituted at Scutari for the reception and distribution of the consignments. Six months after her arrival this was done.

In the meantime, she had reorganised the kitchens and the laundries in the hospitals. The ill-cooked hunks of meat, vilely served at irregular intervals, which had hitherto been the only diet for the sick men, were replaced by punctual meals, well-prepared and appetising, while strengthening extra foods— soups and wines and jellies ('preposterous luxuries', snarled Dr. Hall) —were distributed to those who needed them. One thing, however, she could not effect. The separation of the bones from the meat was no part of official cookery: the rule was that the food must be divided into equal portions, and if some of the portions were all bone— well, every man must take his chance. The rule, perhaps, was not a very good one; but there it was. 'It would require a new Regulation of the Service,' she was told, 'to bone the meat.' As for the washing arrangements, they were revolutionised. Up to the time of Miss Nightingale's arrival, the number of shirts the authorities had succeeded in washing was seven. The hospital bedding, she found, was 'washed' in cold water. She took a Turkish house, had boilers installed, and employed soldiers' wives to do the laundry work. The expenses were defrayed from her own funds and that of The Times; and henceforward, the sick and wounded had the comfort of clean linen.

Then she turned her attention to their clothing. Owing to military exigencies, the greater number of the men had abandoned their kit; their knapsacks were lost forever; they possessed nothing but what was on their persons, and that was usually only fit for speedy destruction. The 'Purveyor', of course, pointed out that, according to the regulations, all soldiers should bring with them into hospital an adequate supply of clothing, and he declared that it was no business of his to make good their deficiencies. Apparently, it was the business of Miss Nightingale. She procured socks, boots, and shirts in enormous quantities; she had trousers made, she rigged up dressing-gowns. 'The fact is,' she told Sidney Herbert, I am now clothing the British Army.'

All at once, word came from the Crimea that a great new contingent of sick and wounded might shortly be expected. Where were they to go? Every available inch in the wards was occupied; the affair was serious and pressing, and the authorities stood aghast. There were some dilapidated rooms in the Barrack Hospital, unfit for human habitation, but Miss Nightingale believed that if measures were promptly taken they might be made capable of accommodating several hundred beds. One of the doctors agreed with her; the rest of the officials were irresolute— it would be a very expensive job, they said; it would involve building; and who could take the responsibility? The proper course was that a representation should be made to the Director-General of the Army Medical Department in London; then the Director-General would apply to the Horse Guards, the Horse Guards would move the Ordnance, the Ordnance would lay the matter before the Treasury, and, if the Treasury gave its consent, the work might be correctly carried through, several months after the necessity for it had disappeared. Miss Nightingale, however, had made up her mind, and she persuaded Lord Stratford— or thought she had persuaded him— to give his sanction to the required expenditure. One hundred and twenty-five workmen were immediately engaged, and the work was begun. The workmen struck; whereupon Lord Stratford washed his hands of the whole business. Miss Nightingale engaged 200 other workmen on her own authority, and paid the bill out of her own resources. The wards were ready by the required date; 500 sick men were received in them; and all the utensils, including knives, forks, spoons, cans and towels, were supplied by Miss Nightingale.

This remarkable woman was in truth performing the function of an administrative chief. How had this come about? Was she not in reality merely a nurse? Was it not her duty simply to tend the sick? And indeed, was it not as a ministering angel, a gentle 'lady with a lamp', that she actually impressed the minds of her contemporaries? No doubt that was so; and yet it is no less certain that, as she herself said, the specific business of nursing was 'the least important of the functions into which she had been forced'. It was clear that in the state of disorganisation into which the hospitals at Scutari had fallen, the most pressing, the really vital, need was for something more than nursing; it was for the necessary elements of civilised life— the commonest material objects, the most ordinary cleanliness, the rudimentary habits of order and authority. 'Oh, dear Miss Nightingale,' said one of her party as they were approaching Constantinople, 'when we land, let there be no delays, let us get straight to nursing the poor fellows!' 'The strongest will be wanted at the wash-tub,' was Miss Nightingale's answer. And it was upon the wash-tub, and all that the wash-tub stood for, that she expended her greatest energies. Yet to say that, is perhaps to say too much. For to those who watched her at work among the sick, moving day and night from bed to bed, with that unflinching courage, with that indefatigable vigilance, it seemed as if the concentrated force of an undivided and unparalleled devotion could hardly suffice for that portion of her task alone.

Wherever, in those vast wards, suffering was at its worst and the need for help was greatest, there, as if by magic, was Miss Nightingale. Her superhuman equanimity would, at the moment of some ghastly operation, nerve the victim to endure, and almost to hope. Her sympathy would assuage the pangs of dying and bring back to those still living something of the forgotten charm of life. Over and over again her untiring efforts rescued those whom the surgeons had abandoned as beyond the possibility of cure. Her mere presence brought with it a strange influence. A passionate idolatry spread among the men— they kissed her shadow as it passed. They did more. 'Before she came,' said a soldier, 'there was cussin' and swearin' but after that it was as 'oly as a church.' The most cherished privilege of the fighting man was abandoned for the sake of Miss Nightingale. In those 'lowest sinks of human misery', as she herself put it, she never heard the use of one expression 'which could distress a gentlewoman'.

She was heroic; and these were the humble tributes paid by those of grosser mould to that high quality. Certainly, she was heroic. Yet her heroism was not of that simple sort so dear to the readers of novels and the compilers of hagiologies— the romantic sentimental heroism with which mankind loves to invest its chosen darlings: it was made of sterner stuff. To the wounded soldier on his couch of agony, she might well appear in the guise of a gracious angel of mercy; but the military surgeons, and the orderlies, and her own nurses, and the 'Purveyor', and Dr. Hall, and, even Lord Stratford himself, could tell a different story. It was not by gentle sweetness and womanly self-abnegation that she had brought order out of chaos in the Scutari hospitals, that, from her own resources, she had clothed the British Army, that she had spread her dominion over the serried and reluctant powers of the official world; it was by strict method, by stern discipline, by rigid attention to detail, by ceaseless labour, and by the fixed determination of an indomitable will.

Beneath her cool and calm demeanour lurked fierce and passionate fires. As she passed through the wards in her plain dress, so quiet, so unassuming, she struck the casual observer simply as the pattern of a perfect lady; but the keener eye perceived something more than that— the serenity of high deliberation in the scope of the capacious brow, the sign of power in the dominating curve of the thin nose, and the traces of a harsh and dangerous temper—something peevish, something mocking, and yet something precise—in the small and delicate mouth. There was humour in the face;

but the curious watcher might wonder whether it was humour of a very pleasant kind; might ask himself, even as he heard the laughter and marked the jokes with which she cheered the spirits of her patients, what sort of sardonic merriment this same lady might not give vent to, in the privacy of her chamber. As for her voice, it was true of it, even more than of her countenance, that it 'had that in it one must fain call master'. Those clear tones were in no need of emphasis: 'I never heard her raise her voice', said one of her companions. 'Only when she had spoken, it seemed as if nothing could follow but obedience.' Once, when she had given some direction, a doctor ventured to remark that the thing could not be done. 'But it must be done,' said Miss Nightingale. A chance bystander, who heard the words, never forgot through all his life the irresistible authority of them. And they were spoken quietly— very quietly indeed.

Late at night, when the long miles of beds lay wrapped in darkness, Miss Nightingale would sit at work in her little room, over her correspondence. It was one of the most formidable of all her duties. There were hundreds of letters to be written to the friends and relations of soldiers; there was the enormous mass of official documents to be dealt with; there were her own private letters to be answered; and, most important of all, there was the composition of her long and confidential reports to Sidney Herbert. These were by no means official communications. Her soul, pent up all day in the restraint and reserve of a vast responsibility, now at last poured itself out in these letters with all its natural vehemence, like a swollen torrent through an open sluice. Here, at least, she did not mince matters. Here she painted in her darkest colours the hideous scenes which surrounded her; here she tore away remorselessly the last veils still shrouding the abominable truth. Then she would fill pages with recommendations and suggestions, with criticisms of the minutest details of organisation, with elaborate calculations of contingencies, with exhaustive analyses and statistical statements piled up in breathless eagerness one on the top of the other. And then her pen, in the virulence of its volubility, would rush on to the discussion of individuals, to the denunciation of an incompetent surgeon or the ridicule of a self- sufficient nurse. Her sarcasm searched the ranks of the officials with the deadly and unsparing precision of a machine-gun. Her nicknames were terrible. She respected no one: Lord Stratford, Lord Raglan, Lady Stratford, Dr. Andrew Smith, Dr. Hall, the Commissary-General, the Purveyor—she fulminated against them all. The intolerable futility of mankind obsessed her like a nightmare, and she gnashed her teeth against it. 'I do well to be angry,' was the burden of her cry. 'How many just men were there at Scutari? How many who cared at all for the sick, or had done anything for their relief? Were there ten? Were there five? Was there even one?' She could not be sure.

At one time, during several weeks, her vituperations descended upon the head of Sidney Herbert himself. He had misinterpreted her wishes, he had traversed her positive instructions, and it was not until he had admitted his error and apologised in abject terms that he was allowed again into favour. While this misunderstanding was at its height, an aristocratic young gentleman arrived at Scutari with a recommendation from the Minister. He had come out from England filled with a romantic desire to render homage to the angelic heroine of his dreams. He had, he said, cast aside his life of ease and luxury; he would devote his days and nights to the service of that gentle lady; he would perform the most menial offices, he would 'fag' for her, he would be her footman— and feel requited by a single smile. A single smile, indeed, he had, but it was of an unexpected kind. Miss Nightingale at first refused to see him, and then, when she consented, believing that he was an emissary sent by Sidney Herbert to put her in the wrong over their dispute, she took notes of her conversation with him, and insisted on his signing them at the end of it. The young gentleman returned to England by the next ship.

This quarrel with Sidney Herbert was, however, an exceptional incident. Alike by him, and by Lord Panmure, his successor at the War Office, she was firmly supported; and the fact that during the whole of her stay at Scutari she had the Home Government at her back, was her trump card in her dealings with the hospital authorities. Nor was it only the Government that was behind her: public opinion in England early recognised the high importance of her mission, and its enthusiastic appreciation of her work soon reached an extraordinary height. The Queen herself was deeply moved. She made repeated inquiries as to the welfare of Miss Nightingale; she asked to see her accounts of the wounded, and made her the intermediary between the throne and the troops. 'Let Mrs. Herbert know,' she wrote to the War Minister, 'that I wish Miss Nightingale and the ladies would tell these poor noble, wounded, and sick men that NO ONE takes a warmer interest or feels MORE for their sufferings or admires their courage and heroism MORE than their Queen. Day and night she thinks of her beloved troops. So does the Prince. Beg Mrs. Herbert to communicate these my words to those ladies, as I know that our sympathy is much valued by these noble fellows.' The letter was read aloud in the wards by the Chaplain. 'It is a very feeling letter,' said the men.

And so the months passed, and that fell winter which had begun with Inkerman and had dragged itself out through the long agony of the investment of Sebastopol, at last was over. In May, 1855, after six months of labour, Miss Nightingale could look with something like satisfaction at the condition of the Scutari hospitals. Had they done nothing more than survive the terrible strain which had been put upon them, it would have been a matter for congratulation; but they had done much more than that— they had marvellously improved. The confusion and the pressure in the wards had come to an end; order reigned in them, and cleanliness; the supplies were bountiful and prompt; important sanitary works had been carried out. One simple comparison of figures was enough

to reveal the extraordinary change: the rate of mortality among the cases treated had fallen from forty-two percent to twenty-two per 1,000. But still, the indefatigable lady was not satisfied. The main problem had been solved— the physical needs of the men had been provided for; their mental and spiritual needs remained. She set up and furnished reading-rooms and recreation rooms. She started classes and lectures. Officers were amazed to see her treating their men as if they were human beings, and assured her that she would only end by 'spoiling the brutes'. But that was not Miss Nightingale's opinion, and she was justified. The private soldier began to drink less and even— though that seemed impossible— to save his pay. Miss Nightingale became a banker for the Army, receiving and sending home large sums of money every month. At last, reluctantly, the Government followed suit, and established machinery of its own for the remission of money.Lord Panmure, however, remained sceptical; 'it will do no good,' he pronounced; 'the British soldier is not a remitting animal.' But, in fact during the next six months £71,000 was sent home.

Amid all these activities, Miss Nightingale took up the further task of inspecting the hospitals in the Crimea itself. The labour was extreme, and the conditions of life were almost intolerable. She spent whole days in the saddle, or was driven over those bleak and rocky heights in a baggage cart. Sometimes she stood for hours in the heavily failing snow, and would only reach her hut at dead of night after walking for miles through perilous ravines. Her powers of resistance seemed incredible, but at last they were exhausted. She was attacked by fever, and for a moment came very near to death. Yet she worked on; if she could not move, she could at least write, and write she did until her mind had left her; and after it had left her, in what seemed the delirious trance of death itself, she still wrote. When, after many weeks, she was strong enough to travel, she was implored to return to England, but she utterly refused. She would not go back, she said, before the last of the soldiers had left Scutari.

This happy moment had almost arrived, when suddenly the smouldering hostilities of the medical authorities burst out into a flame. Dr. Hall's labours had been rewarded by a K.C.B— letters which, as Miss Nightingale told Sidney Herbert, she could only suppose to mean 'Knight of the Crimean Burial-Grounds'— and the honour had turned his head. He was Sir John, and he would be thwarted no longer. Disputes had lately arisen between Miss Nightingale and some of the nurses in the Crimean hospitals. The situation had been embittered by rumours of religious dissensions, while the Crimean nurses were Roman Catholics, many of those at Scutari were suspected of a regrettable propensity towards the tenets of Dr. Pusey. Miss Nightingale was by no means disturbed by these sectarian differences, but any suggestion that her supreme authority over all the nurses with the Army was, no doubt, enough to rouse her to fury; and it appeared that Mrs. Bridgeman, the Reverend Mother in the Crimea, had ventured to call that authority in question. Sir John Hall thought that his opportunity had come, and strongly supported Mrs. Bridgeman— or, as Miss Nightingale preferred to call her, the 'Reverend Brickbat'.

There was a violent struggle; Miss Nightingale's rage was terrible. Dr. Hall, she declared, was doing his best to 'root her out of the Crimea'. She would bear it no longer; the War Office was playing her false; there was only one thing to be done— Sidney Herbert must move for the production of papers in the House of Commons, so that the public might be able to judge between her and her enemies. Sidney Herbert, with great difficulty, calmed her down. Orders were immediately dispatched putting her supremacy beyond doubt, and the Reverend Brickbat withdrew from the scene. Sir John, however, was more tenacious. A few weeks later, Miss Nightingale and her nurses visited the Crimea for the last time, and the brilliant idea occurred to him that he could crush her by a very simple expedient— he would starve her into submission; and he actually ordered that no rations of any kind should be supplied to her. He had already tried this plan with great effect upon an unfortunate medical man whose presence in the Crimea he had considered an intrusion; but he was now to learn that such tricks were thrown away upon Miss Nightingale. With extraordinary foresight, she had brought with her a great supply of food; she succeeded in obtaining more at her own expense and by her own exertions; and thus for ten days, in that inhospitable country, she was able to feed herself and twenty-four nurses. Eventually, the military authorities intervened in her favour, and Sir John had to confess that he was beaten.

It was not until July, 1856—four months after the Declaration of Peace— that Miss Nightingale left Scutari for England. Her reputation was now enormous, and the enthusiasm of the public was unbounded. The royal approbation was expressed by the gift of a brooch, accompanied by a private letter. 'You are, I know, well aware,' wrote Her Majesty, 'of the high sense I entertain of the Christian devotion which you have displayed during this great and bloody war, and I need hardly repeat to you how warm my admiration is for your services, which are fully equal to those of my dear and brave soldiers, whose sufferings you have had the privilege of alleviating in so merciful a manner. I am, however, anxious of marking my feelings in a manner which I trust will be agreeable to you, and therefore, send you with this letter a brooch, the form and emblems of which commemorate your great and blessed work, and which I hope you will wear as a mark of the high approbation of your Sovereign!

'It will be a very great satisfaction to me,' Her Majesty added, 'to make the acquaintance of one who has set so bright an example to our sex.'

The brooch, which was designed by the Prince Consort, bore a St . George's cross in red enamel, and the Royal cipher surmounted by diamonds. The whole was encircled by the inscription 'Blessed are the Merciful'.

III

THE name of Florence Nightingale lives in the memory of the world by virtue of the lurid and heroic adventure of the Crimea. Had she died—as she nearly did—upon her return to England, her reputation would hardly have been different; her legend would have come down to us almost as we know it today—that gentle vision of female virtue which first took shape before the adoring eyes of the sick soldiers at Scutari. Yet, as a matter of fact, she lived for more than half a century after the Crimean War; and during the greater part of that long period, all the energy and all the devotion of her extraordinary nature were working at their highest pitch. What she accomplished in those years of unknown labour could, indeed, hardly have been more glorious than her Crimean triumphs, but it was certainly more important. The true history was far stranger even than the myth. In Miss Nightingale's own eyes the adventure of the Crimea was a mere incident— scarcely more than a useful stepping-stone in her career. It was the fulcrum with which she hoped to move the world; but it was only the fulcrum. For more than a generation she was to sit in secret, working her lever: and her real "life" began at the very moment when, in the popular imagination, it had ended.

She arrived in England in a shattered state of health. The hardships and the ceaseless effort of the last two years had undermined her nervous system; her heart was pronounced to be affected; she suffered constantly from fainting-fits and terrible attacks of utter physical prostration. The doctors declared that one thing alone would save her— a complete and prolonged rest. But that was also the one thing with which she would have nothing to do. She had never been in the habit of resting; why should she begin now? Now, when her opportunity had come at last; now, when the iron was hot, and it was time to strike? No; she had work to do; and, come what might, she would do it. The doctors protested in vain; in vain her family lamented and entreated; in vain her friends pointed out to her the madness of such a course. Madness? Mad—possessed—perhaps she was. A demoniac frenzy had seized upon her. As she lay upon her sofa, gasping, she devoured blue- books, dictated letters, and, in the intervals of her palpitations, cracked her febrile jokes. For months at a stretch she never left her bed. For years she was in daily expectation of death. But she would not rest. At this rate, the doctors assured her, even if she did not die, she would, become an invalid for life. She could not help that; there was the work to be done; and, as for rest, very likely she might rest ... when she had done it.

Wherever she went, in London or in the country, in the hills of Derbyshire, or among the rhododendrons at Embley, she was haunted by a ghost. It was the spectre of Scutari— the hideous vision of the organisation of a military hospital. She would lay that phantom, or she would perish. The whole system of the Army Medical Department, the education of the Medical Officer, the regulations of hospital procedure ... REST? How could she rest while these things were as they were, while, if the like necessity were to arise again, the like results would follow? And, even in peace and at home, what was the sanitary condition of the Army? The mortality in the barracks was, she found, nearly double the mortality in civil life. 'You might as well take 1,100 men every year out upon Salisbury Plain and shoot them,' she said. After inspecting the hospitals at Chatham, she smiled grimly. 'Yes, this is one more symptom of the system which, in the Crimea, put to death 16,000 men.' Scutari had given her knowledge; and it had given her power too: her enormous reputation was at her back— an incalculable force. Other work, other duties, might lie before her; but the most urgent, the most obvious of all, was to look to the health of the Army.

One of her very first steps was to take advantage of the invitation which Queen Victoria had sent her to the Crimea, together with the commemorative brooch. Within a few weeks of her return she visited Balmoral, and had several interviews with both the Queen and the Prince, Consort. 'She put before us,' wrote the Prince in his diary, 'all the defects of our present military hospital system, and the reforms that are needed.' She related 'the whole story' of her experiences in the East; and, in addition, she managed to have some long and confidential talks with His Royal Highness on metaphysics and religion. The impression which she created was excellent. 'Sie gefällt uns sehr,' noted the Prince, 'ist sehr bescheiden.' Her Majesty's comment was different—'Such a HEAD! I wish we had her at the War Office.'

But Miss Nightingale was not at the War Office, and for a very simple reason: she was a woman. Lord Panmure, however, was (though indeed the reason for that was not quite so simple); and it was upon Lord Panmure that the issue of Miss Nightingale's efforts for reform must primarily depend. That burly Scottish nobleman had not, in spite of his most earnest endeavours, had a very easy time of it as Secretary of State for War. He had come into office in the middle of the SebastopolCampaign, and had felt himself very well fitted for the position, since he had acquired in former days an inside knowledge of the Army—as a Captain of Hussars. It was this inside knowledge which had enabled him to inform Miss Nightingale with such authority that 'the British soldier is not a remitting animal'. And perhaps it was this same consciousness of a command of his subject which had impelled him to write a dispatch to Lord Raglan, blandly informing the Commander-in-Chief in the Field just how he was neglecting his duties, and pointing out to him that if he would only try he really might do a little better next time.

Lord Raglan's reply, calculated as it was to make its recipient sink into the earth, did not quite have that effect upon Lord Panmure, who, whatever might have been his faults, had never been accused of being supersensitive. However, he allowed the matter to drop; and a little later Lord Raglan died—worn out, some people said, by work and anxiety. He was succeeded by an excellent red-nosed old gentleman, General Simpson, whom nobody has ever heard of, and who took Sebastopol. But Lord Panmure's relations with him were hardly more satisfactory than his relations with Lord Raglan; for, while Lord Raglan had been too independent, poor General Simpson erred in the opposite direction, perpetually asked advice, suffered from lumbago, doubted (his nose growingredder and redder daily) whether he was fit for his post, and, by alternate mails, sent in and withdrew his resignation. Then, too, both the General and the Minister suffered acutely from that distressingly useful new invention, the electric telegraph. On one occasion General Simpson felt obliged actually to expostulate. 'I think, my Lord,' he wrote, 'that some telegraphic messages reach us that cannot be sent under due authority, and are perhaps unknown to you, although under the protection of your Lordship's name.

For instance, I was called up last night, a dragoon having come express with a telegraphic message in these words, "Lord Panmure to General Simpson—Captain Jarvis has been bitten by a centipede. How is he now?"' General Simpson might have put up with this, though to be sure it did seem 'rather too trifling an affair to call for a dragoon to ride a couple of miles in the dark that he may knock up the Commander of the Army out of the very small allowance of sleep permitted; but what was really more than he could bear was to find 'upon sending in the morning another mounted dragoon to inquire after Captain Jarvis, four miles off, that he never has been bitten at all, but has had a boil, from which he is fast recovering'. But Lord Panmure had troubles of his own. His favourite nephew, Captain Dowbiggin, was at the front, and to one of his telegrams to the Commander-in- Chief the Minister had taken occasion to append the following carefully qualified sentence—'I recommend Dowbiggin to your notice, should you have a vacancy, and if he is fit'. Unfortunately, in those early days, it was left to the discretion of the telegraphist to compress the messages which passed through his hands; so that the result was that Lord Panmure's delicate appeal reached its destination in the laconic form of 'Look after Dowb'. The Headquarters Staff were at first extremely puzzled; they were at last extremely amused. The story spread; and 'Look after Dowb' remained for many years the familiar formula for describing official hints in favour of deserving nephews.

And now that all this was over, now that Sebastopol had been, somehow or another, taken; now that peace was, somehow or another, made; now that the troubles of office might surely be expected to be at an end at last— here was Miss Nightingale breaking in upon the scene with her talk about the state of the hospitals and the necessity for sanitary reform. It was most irksome; and Lord Panmure almost began to wish that he was engaged upon some more congenial occupation—discussing, perhaps, the constitution of the Free Church of Scotland—a question in which he was profoundly interested. But no; duty was paramount; and he set himself, with a sigh of resignation, to the task of doing as little of it as he possibly could.

'The Bison' his friends called him; and the name fitted both his physical demeanour and his habit of mind. That large low head seemed to have been created for butting rather than for anything else. There he stood, four-square and menacing in the doorway of reform; and it remained to be seen whether, the bulky mass, upon whose solid hide even the barbed arrows of Lord Raglan's scorn had made no mark, would prove amenable to the pressure of Miss Nightingale. Nor was he alone in the doorway. There loomed behind him the whole phalanx of professional conservatism, the stubborn supporters of the out-of-date, the worshippers and the victims of War Office routine. Among these it was only natural that Dr. Andrew Smith, the head

of the Army Medical Department, should have been
pre-eminent—Dr. Andrew Smith, who had assured
Miss Nightingale before she left England that
'nothing was wanted at Scutari'. Such were her
opponents; but she too was not without allies. She
had gained the ear of Royalty—which was
something; at any moment that she pleased she
could gain the ear of the public—which was a great
deal. She had a host of admirers and friends;
and—to say nothing of her personal qualities—her
knowledge, her tenacity, her tact—she possessed,
too, one advantage which then, far more even than
now, carried an immense weight— she belonged to
the highest circle of society. She moved naturally
among Peers and Cabinet Ministers—she was one of
their own set; and in those days their set was a very
narrow one. What kind of attention would such
persons have paid to some middle-class woman with
whom they were not acquainted, who possessed
great experience of Army nursing and had decided
views upon hospital reform? They would have
politely ignored her; but it was impossible to ignore
Flo Nightingale. When she spoke, they were obliged
to listen; and, when they had once begun to do
that— what might not follow? She knew her power,
and she used it. She supported her weightiest
minutes with familiar witty little notes. The Bison
began to look grave. It might be difficult—it might
be damned difficult—to put down one's head against
the white hand of a lady...

Of Miss Nightingale's friends, the most important
was Sidney Herbert. He was a man upon whom the
good fairies seemed to have showered, as he lay in
his cradle, all their most enviable goods. Well born,
handsome, rich, the master of Wilton—one of those
great country-houses, clothed with the glamour of a

historic past, which are the peculiar glory of England—he possessed— besides all these advantages: so charming, so lively, so gentle a disposition that no one who had once come near him could ever be his enemy.

He was, in fact, a man of whom it was difficult not to say that he was a perfect English gentleman. For his virtues were equal even to his good fortune. He was religious, deeply religious. 'I am more and more convinced every day,' he wrote, when he had been for some years a Cabinet Minister, 'that in politics, as in everything else, nothing can be right which is not in accordance with the spirit of the Gospel.' No one was more unselfish; he was charitable and benevolent to a remarkable degree; and he devoted the whole of his life, with an unwavering conscientiousness, to the public service. With such a character, with such opportunities, what high hopes must have danced before him, what radiant visions of accomplished duties, of ever-increasing usefulness, of beneficent power, of the consciousness of disinterested success! Some of those hopes and visions were, indeed, realised; but, in the end, the career of Sidney Herbert seemed to show that, with all their generosity, there was some gift or other— what was it?—some essential gift—which the good fairies had withheld, and that even the qualities of a perfect English gentleman may be no safeguard against anguish, humiliation, and defeat.

That career would certainly have been very different if he had never known Miss Nightingale. The alliance between them which had begun with her appointment to Scutari, which had grown closer and closer while the war lasted, developed, after her return, into one of the most extraordinary friendships. It was the friendship of a man and a woman intimately bound together by their devotion to a public cause; mutual affection, of course, played a part in it, but it was an incidental part; the whole soul of the relationship was a community of work. Perhaps out of England such an intimacy could hardly have existed—an intimacy so utterly untinctured not only by passion itself but by the suspicion of it. For years Sidney Herbert saw Miss Nightingale almost daily, for long hours together, corresponding with her incessantly when they were apart; and the tongue of scandal was silent; and one of the most devoted of her admirers was his wife. But what made the connection still more remarkable was the way in which the parts that were played in it were divided between the two. The man who acts, decides, and achieves; the woman who encourages, applauds, and—from a distance—inspires: the combination is common enough; but Miss Nightingale was neither an Aspasia nor an Egeria. In her case it is almost true to say that the roles were reversed; the qualities of pliancy and sympathy fell to the man, those of command and initiative to the woman.

There was one thing only which Miss Nightingale lacked in her equipment for public life; she had not— she never could have— the public power and authority which belonged to the successful politician. That power and authority Sidney Herbert possessed; that fact was obvious, and the conclusions no less so: it was through the man that the woman must work her will. She took hold of him, taught him, shaped him, absorbed him, dominated him through and through. He did not resist—he did not wish to resist; his natural inclination lay along the same path as hers; only that terrific personality swept him forward at her own fierce pace and with her own relentless stride. Swept him—where to? Ah! Why had he ever known Miss Nightingale? If Lord Panmure was a bison, Sidney Herbert, no doubt, was a stag— a comely, gallant creature springing through the forest; but the forest is a dangerous place. One has the image of those wide eyes fascinated suddenly by something feline, something strong; there is a pause; and then the tigress has her claws in the quivering haunches; and then—!

Besides Sidney Herbert, she had other friends who, in a more restricted sphere, were hardly less essential to her. If, in her condition of bodily collapse, she were to accomplish what she was determined that she should accomplish, the attentions and the services of others would be absolutely indispensable. Helpers and servers she must have; and accordingly there was soon formed about her a little group of devoted disciples upon whose affections and energies she could implicitly rely. Devoted, indeed, these disciples were, in no ordinary sense of the term; for certainly she was no light taskmistress, and he who set out to be of use to Miss Nightingale was apt to find, before he had gone very far, that he was in truth being made use of in good earnest to the very limit of his endurance and his capacity. Perhaps, even beyond those limits; why not? Was she asking of others more than she was giving herself? Let them look at her lying there pale and breathless on the couch; could it be said that she spared herself? Why, then, should she spare others? And it was not for her own sake that she made these claims. For her own sake, indeed! No! They all knew it! it was for the sake of the work. And so the little band, bound body and soul in that strange servitude, laboured on ungrudgingly.

Among the most faithful was her 'Aunt Mai', her
father's sister, who from the earliest days had stood
beside her, who had helped her to escape from the
thraldom of family life, who had been with her at
Scutari, and who now acted almost the part of a
mother to her, watching over her with infinite care
in all the movements and uncertainties which her
state of health involved. Another constant attendant
was her brother-in-law, Sir Harry Verney, whom she
found particularly valuable in parliamentary affairs.
Arthur Clough, the poet, also a connection by
marriage, she used in other ways. Ever since he had
lost his faith at the time of the Oxford Movement,
Clough had passed his life in a condition of
considerable uneasiness, which was increased rather
than diminished by the practice of poetry. Unable to
decide upon the purpose of an existence whose
savour had fled together with his belief in the
Resurrection, his spirits lowered still further by
ill-health, and his income not all that it should be, he
had determined to seek the solution of his difficulties
in the United States of America. But, even there, the
solution was not forthcoming; and, when, a little
later, he was offered a post in a government
department at home, he accepted it, came to live in
London, and immediately fell under the influence of
Miss Nightingale. Though the purpose of existence
might be still uncertain and its nature still
unsavoury, here, at any rate, under the eye of this
inspired woman, was something real, something
earnest: his only doubt was— could he be of any use?
Certainly he could. There were a great number of
miscellaneous little jobs which there was nobody
handy to do. For instance, when Miss Nightingale
was travelling, there were the railway- tickets to be
taken; and there were proof-sheets to be corrected;

and then there were parcels to be done up in brown paper, and carried to the post. Certainly he could be useful. And so, upon such occupations as these, Arthur Clough was set to work. 'This that I see, is not all,' he comforted himself by reflecting, 'and this that I do is but little; nevertheless it is good, though there is better than it.'As time went on, her 'Cabinet', as she called it, grew larger. Officials with whom her work brought her into touch and who sympathised with her objects, were pressed into her service; and old friends of the Crimean days gathered around her when they returned to England. Among these the most indefatigable was Dr. Sutherland, a sanitary expert, who for more than thirty years acted as her confidential private secretary, and surrendered to her purposes literally the whole of his life. Thus sustained and assisted, thus slaved for and adored, she prepared to beard the Bison.

Two facts soon emerged, and all that followed turned upon them. It became clear, in the first place, that that imposing mass was not immovable, and, in the second, that its movement, when it did move, would be exceeding slow. The Bison was no match for the Lady. It was in vain that he put down his head and planted his feet in the earth; he could not withstand her; the white hand forced him back. But the process was an extraordinarily gradual one. Dr. Andrew Smith and all his War Office phalanx stood behind, blocking the way; the poor Bison groaned inwardly, and cast a wistful eye towards the happy pastures of the Free Church of Scotland; then slowly, with infinite reluctance, step by step, he retreated, disputing every inch of the ground.

The first great measure, which, supported as it was by the Queen, the Cabinet, and the united opinion of the country, it was impossible to resist, was the appointment of a Royal Commission to report upon the health of the Army. The question of the composition of the Commission then immediately arose; and it was over this matter that the first hand-to-hand encounter between Lord Panmure and Miss Nightingale took place. They met, and Miss Nightingale was victorious; Sidney Herbert was appointed Chairman; and, in the end, the only member of the Commission opposed to her views was Dr. Andrew Smith. During the interview, Miss Nightingale made an important discovery: she found that 'the Bison was bullyable'—the hide was the hide of a Mexican buffalo, but the spirit was the spirit of an Alderney calf. And there was one thing above all others which the huge creature dreaded—an appeal to public opinion. The faintest hint of such a terrible eventuality made his heart dissolve within him; he would agree to anything he would cut short his grouse-shooting—he would make a speech in the House of Lords, he would even overrule Dr. Andrew Smith—rather than that. Miss Nightingale held the fearful threat in reserve—she would speak out what she knew; she would publish the truth to the whole world, and let the whole world judge between them. With supreme skill, she kept this sword of Damocles

poised above the Bison's head, and more than once she was actually on the point of really dropping it— for his recalcitrancy grew and grew.

The personnel of the Commission once determined upon, there was a struggle, which lasted for six months, over the nature of its powersWas it to be an efficient body, armed with the right of full inquiry and wide examination, or was it to be a polite official contrivance for exonerating Dr.

Andrew Smith? The War Office phalanx closed its ranks, and fought tooth and nail; but it was defeated: the Bison was bullyable. 'Three months from this day,' Miss Nightingale had written at last, 'I publish my experience of the Crimean Campaign, and my suggestions for improvement, unless there has been a fair and tangible pledge by that time for reform.' Who could face that?

And, if the need came, she meant to be as good as her word. For she had now determined, whatever might be the fate of the Commission, to draw up her own report upon the questions at issue. The labour involved was enormous; her health was almost desperate; but she did not flinch, and after six months of incredible industry she had put together and written with her own hand her Notes affecting the Health, Efficiency, and Hospital Administration of the British Army. This extraordinary composition, filling more than 800 closely printed pages, laying down vast principles of far-reaching reform, discussing the minutest details of a multitude of controversial subjects, containing an enormous mass of information of the most varied kinds—military, statistical, sanitary, architectural—was never given to the public, for the need never came; but it formed the basis of the Report of the Royal Commission; and it remains to this day the leading authority on the medical administration of armies.

Before it had been completed, the struggle over the powers of the Commission had been brought to a victorious close. Lord Panmure had given way once more; he had immediately hurried to the Queen to obtain her consent; and only then, when Her Majesty's initials had been irrevocably affixed to the fatal document, did he dare to tell Dr. Andrew Smith what he had done. The Commission met, and another immense load fell upon Miss Nightingale's shoulders. Today she would, of course, have been one of the Commission herself; but at that time the idea of a woman appearing in such a capacity was unheard of; and no one even suggested the possibility of Miss Nightingale's doing so. The result was that she was obliged to remain behind the scenes throughout, to coach Sidney Herbert in private at every important juncture, and to convey to him and to her other friends upon the Commission the vast funds of her expert knowledge—so essential in the examination of witnesses—by means of innumerable consultations, letters, and memoranda. It was even doubtful whether the proprieties would admit of her giving evidence; and at last, as a compromise, her modesty only allowed her to do so in the form of written answers to written questions. At length, the grand affair was finished. The Commission's Report, embodying almost word for word the suggestions of Miss Nightingale, was drawn up by Sidney Herbert. Only one question remained to be answered—would anything, after all, be done? Or would the Royal Commission, like so many other Royal Commissions before and since, turn out to have achieved nothing but the concoction of a very fat bluebook on a very high shelf?

And so the last and the deadliest struggle with the Bison began. Six months had been spent in coercing him into granting the Commission effective powers; six more months were occupied by the work of the Commission; and now yet another six were to pass in extorting from him the means whereby the recommendations of the Commission might be actually carried out. But, in the end, the thing was done. Miss Nightingale seemed, indeed, during these months, to be upon the very brink of death. Accompanied by the faithful Aunt Mai, she moved from place to place—to Hampstead, to Highgate, to Derbyshire, to Malvern—in what appeared to be a last desperate effort to find health somewhere; but she carried that with her which made health impossible. Her desire for work could now scarcely be distinguished from mania. At one moment she was writing a 'last letter' to Sidney Herbert; at the next she was offering to go out to India to nurse the sufferers in the Mutiny. When Dr. Sutherland wrote, imploring her to take a holiday, she raved. Rest!—'I am lying without my head, without my claws, and you all peck at me. It is de rigueur, d'obligation, like the saying something to one's hat, when one goes into church, to say to me all that has been said to me 110 times a day during the last three months. It is the obbligato on the violin, and the twelve violins all practise it together, like the clocks striking twelve o'clock at night all over London, till I say like Xavier de Maistre, Assez, je sais, je ne le sais que trop. I am not a penitent; but you are like the R.C. confessor, who says what is de rigueur. ...'

Her wits began to turn, and there was no holding her. She worked like a slave in a mine. She began to believe, as she had begun to believe at Scutari, that none of her fellow-workers had their hearts in the business; if they had, why did they not work as she did? She could only see slackness and stupidity around her. Dr. Sutherland, of course, was grotesquely muddle-headed; and Arthur Clough incurably lazy. Even Sidney Herbert ... oh yes, he had simplicity and candour and quickness of perception, no doubt; but he was an eclectic; and what could one hope for from a man who went away to fish in Ireland just when the Bison most needed bullying? As for the Bison himself, he had fled to Scotland where he remained buried for many months. The fate of the vital recommendation in the Commission's Report—the appointment of four Sub-Commissions charged with the duty of determining upon the details of the proposed reforms and of putting them into execution—still hung in the balance. The Bison consented to everything; and then, on a flying visit to London, withdrew his consent and hastily returned to Scotland. Then for many weeks all business was suspended; he had gout—gout in the hands— so that he could not write. 'His gout was always handy,' remarked Miss Nightingale. But eventually it was clear even to the Bison that the game was up, and the inevitable surrender came.

There was, however, one point in which he triumphed over Miss Nightingale: the building of Netley Hospital had been begun under his orders, before her return to England. Soon after her arrival she examined the plans, and found that they reproduced all the worst faults of an out-of-date and mischievous system of hospital construction. She therefore urged that the matter should be reconsidered, and in the meantime the building stopped. But the Bison was obdurate; it would be very expensive, and in any case it was too late. Unable to make any impression on him, and convinced of the extreme importance of the question, she determined to appeal to a higher authority. Lord Palmerston was Prime Minister; she had known him from her childhood; he was a near neighbour of her father's in the New Forest. She went down to the New Forest, armed with the plan of the proposed hospital and all the relevant information, stayed the night at Lord Palmerston's house, and convinced him of the necessity of rebuilding Netley. 'It seems to me,' Lord Palmerston wrote to Lord Panmure, 'that at Netley all consideration of what would best tend to the comfort and recovery of the patients has been sacrificed to the vanity of the architect, whose sole object has been to make a building which should cut a dash when looked at from the Southampton river... Pray, therefore, stop all further progress in the work until the matter can be duly considered.' But the Bison was not to be moved by one peremptory letter, even if it was from the Prime Minister. He put forth all his powers of procrastination, Lord Palmerston lost interest in the subject, and so the chief military hospital in England was triumphantly completed on insanitary principles, with unventilated rooms, and with all the patients' windows facing northeast.

But now the time had come when the Bison was to trouble and to be troubled no more. A vote in the House of Commons brought about the fall of Lord Palmerston's Government, and, Lord Panmure found himself at liberty to devote the rest of his life to the Free Church of Scotland. After a brief interval, Sidney Herbert became Secretary of State for War. Great was the jubilation in the Nightingale Cabinet: the day of achievement had dawned at last. The next two and a half years (1859-61) saw the introduction of the whole system of reforms for which Miss Nightingale had been struggling so fiercely—reforms which make Sidney Herbert's tenure of power at the War Office an important epoch in the history of the British Army. The four Sub-Commissions, firmly established under the immediate control of the Minister, and urged forward by the relentless perseverance of Miss Nightingale, set to work with a will. The barracks and the hospitals were remodelled; they were properly ventilated and warmed and lighted for the first time; they were given a water supply which actually supplied water, and kitchens where, strange to say, it was possible to cook. Then the great question of the Purveyor—that portentous functionary whose powers and whose lack of powers had weighed like a nightmare upon Scutari—was taken in hand, and new regulations were laid down, accurately defining his responsibilities and his duties. One Sub-Commission reorganised the medical statistics of the Army; another established in spite of the last convulsive efforts of the Department an Army Medical School. Finally, the Army Medical Department itself was completely reorganised; an administrative code was drawn up; and the great and novel principle was established that it was as much a part of the duty of the authorities to look after the soldier's health as to look after his sickness. Besides this, it was at last officially admitted that he had a moral and intellectual side. Coffee-rooms and reading-rooms, gymnasiums and workshops were instituted. A new era did in truth appear to have begun. Already by 1861 the mortality in the Army had decreased by one- half since the days of the Crimea. It was no wonder that even vaster possibilities began now to open out before Miss Nightingale. One thing was still needed to complete and to assure her triumphs. The Army Medical Department was indeed reorganised; but the great central machine was still untouched. The War Office itself—! If she could remould that nearer to her heart's desire- -there indeed would be a victory! And until that final act was accomplished, how could she be certain that all the rest of her achievements might not, by some capricious turn of Fortune's wheel—a change of

Ministry, perhaps, replacing Sidney Herbert by some puppet of the permanent official gang— be swept to limbo in a moment?

Meanwhile, still ravenous for yet more and more work, her activities had branched out into new directions. The Army in India claimed her attention. A Sanitary Commission, appointed at her suggestion, and working under her auspices, did for our troops there what the four Sub-Commissions were doing for those at home. At the same time, these very years which saw her laying the foundations of the whole modern system of medical work in the Army, saw her also beginning to bring her knowledge, her influence, and her activity into the service of the country at large. Her "Notes on Hospitals" (1859) revolutionised the theory of hospital construction and hospital management. She was immediately recognised as the leading expert upon all the questions involved; her advice flowed unceasingly and in all directions, so that there is no great hospital today which does not bear upon it the impress of her mind. Nor was this all. With the opening of the Nightingale Training School for Nurses at St. Thomas's Hospital (1860), she became the founder of modern nursing.

But a terrible crisis was now fast approaching. Sidney Herbert had consented to undertake the root and branch reform of the War Office. He had sallied forth into that tropical jungle of festooned obstructiveness, of intertwisted irresponsibilities, of crouching prejudices, of abuses grown stiff and rigid with antiquity, which for so many years to come was destined to lure reforming Ministers to their doom. 'The War Office,' said Miss Nightingale, 'is a very slow office, an enormously expensive office, and one in which the Minister's intentions can be entirely negated by all his sub-departments, and those of each of the sub-departments by every other.' It was true; and of course, at the, first rumour of a change, the old phalanx of reaction was bristling with its accustomed spears. At its head stood no longer Dr. Andrew Smith, who, some time since, had followed the Bison into outer darkness, but a yet more formidable figure, the Permanent Under-Secretary himself, Sir Benjamin Hawes— Ben Hawes the Nightingale Cabinet irreverently dubbed him "a man remarkable even among civil servants for adroitness in baffling inconvenient inquiries, resource in raising false issues, and, in, short, a consummate command of all the arts of officially sticking in the mud'.

'Our scheme will probably result in Ben Hawes's resignation,' Miss Nightingale said; 'and that is another of its advantages.' Ben Hawes himself, however, did not quite see it in that light. He set himself to resist the wishes of the Minister by every means in his power. The struggle was long, and desperate; and, as it proceeded, it gradually became evident to Miss Nightingale that something was the matter with Sidney Herbert. What was it? His health, never very strong, was, he said, in danger of collapsing under the strain of his work. But, after all, what is illness, when there is a War Office to be reorganised? Then he began to talk of retiring altogether from public life. The doctors were consulted, and declared that, above all things, what was necessary was rest. Rest! She grew seriously alarmed. Was it possible that, at the last moment, the crowning wreath of victory was to be snatched from her grasp? She was not to be put aside by doctors; they were talking nonsense; the necessary thing was not rest, but the reform of the War Office;

and, besides, she knew very well from her own case what one could do even when one was on the point of death.

She expostulated vehemently, passionately; the goal was so near, so very near; he could not turn back now! At any rate, he could not resist Miss Nightingale. A compromise was arranged. Very reluctantly, he exchanged the turmoil of the House of Commons for the dignity of the House of Lords, and he remained at the War Office. She was delighted. 'One fight more, the best and the last,' she said.

For several more months the fight did indeed go on. But the strain upon him was greater even than she perhaps could realise. Besides the intestine war in his office, he had to face a constant battle in the Cabinet with Mr. Gladstone—a more redoubtable antagonist even than Ben Hawes—over the estimates. His health grew worse and worse. He was attacked by faintingfits; and there were some days when he could only just keep himself going by gulps of brandy. Miss Nightingale spurred him forward with her encouragements and her admonitions, her zeal and her example. But at last his spirit began to sink as well as his body. He could no longer hope; he could no longer desire; it was useless, all useless; it was utterly impossible. He had failed. The dreadful moment came when the truth was forced upon him: he would never be able to reform the War Office. But a yet more dreadful moment lay behind; he must go to Miss Nightingale and tell her that he was a failure, a beaten man.

'Blessed are the merciful!' What strange ironic prescience had led Prince Albert, in the simplicity of his heart, to choose that motto for the Crimean brooch? The words hold a double lesson; and, alas!

when she brought herself to realise at length what was indeed the fact and what there was no helping, it was not in mercy that she turned upon her old friend.

'Beaten!' she exclaimed. 'Can't you see that you've simply thrown away the game? And with all the winning cards in your hands! And so noble a game! Sidney Herbert beaten! And beaten by Ben Hawes! It is a worse disgrace...' her full rage burst out at last, '...a worse disgrace than the hospitals at Scutari.'

He dragged himself away from her, dragged himself to Spa, hoping vainly for a return to health, and then, despairing, back again to England, to Wilton, to the majestic house standing there resplendent in the summer sunshine, among the great cedars which had lent their shade to Sir Philip Sidney, and all those familiar, darling haunts of beauty which he loved, each one of them, 'as if they were persons'; and at, Wilton he died. After having received the Eucharist, he had become perfectly calm; then, almost unconscious, his lips were seen to be moving. Those about him bent down. 'Poor Florence! Poor Florence!' they just caught. '...Our joint work ... unfinished ... tried to do ...' and they could hear no more.

When the onward rush of a powerful spirit sweeps a weaker one to its destruction, the commonplaces of the moral judgment are better left unmade. If Miss Nightingale had been less ruthless, Sidney Herbert would not have perished; but then, she would not have been Miss Nightingale. The force that created was the force that destroyed. It was her Demon that was responsible. When the fatal news reached her, she was overcome by agony. In the revulsion of her feelings, she made a worship of the dead man's memory; and the facile instrument which had broken in her hand she spoke of forever after as her 'Master'. Then, almost at the same moment, another blow fell on her. Arthur Clough, worn out by labours very different from those of Sidney Herbert, died too: never more would he tie up her parcels. And yet a thirddisaster followed. The faithful Aunt Mai did not, to be sure, die; no, she did something almost worse: she left Miss Nightingale. She was growing old, and she felt that she had closer and more imperative duties with her own family. Her niece could hardly forgive her. She poured out, in one of her enormous letters, a passionate diatribe upon the faithlessness, the lack of sympathy, the stupidity, the ineptitude of women. Her doctrines had taken no hold among them; she had never known one who had appris a apprendre; she could not even get a woman secretary; 'they don't know the names of the Cabinet Ministers—they don't know which of the Churches has Bishops and which not'. As for the spirit of self-sacrifice, well—Sidney Herbert and Arthur Clough were men, and they indeed had shown their devotion; but women—! She would mount three widow's caps 'for a sign'. The first two would be for Clough and for her Master; but the third—'the biggest widow's cap of all'—would be for Aunt Mai. She did well to be angry; she was deserted in her hour of need; and after all, could she be sure that even the male sex was so impeccable? There was Dr. Sutherland, bungling as usual. Perhaps even he intended to go off one of these days, too? She gave him a look, and he shivered in his shoes. No!—she grinned sardonically; she would always have Dr. Sutherland. And then she reflected that there was one thing more that she would always have— her work.

IV

SIDNEY HERBERT'S death finally put an end to
Miss Nightingale's dream of a reformed War Office.
For a moment, indeed, in the first agony of her
disappointment, she had wildly clutched at a straw;
she had written to M. Gladstone to beg him to take
up the burden of Sidney Herbert's work. And Mr.
Gladstone had replied with a sympathetic account of
the funeral.

Succeeding Secretaries of State managed
between them to undo a good deal of what had been
accomplished, but they could not undo it all; and for
ten years more (1862-72) Miss Nightingale
remained a potent influence at the War Office. After
that, her direct connection with the Army came to an
end, and her energies began to turn more and more
completely towards more general objects. Her work
upon hospital reform assumed enormous
proportions; she was able to improve the conditions
in infirmaries and workhouses; and one of her most
remarkable papers forestalls the recommendations
of the Poor Law Commission of 1909. Her training,
school for nurses, with all that it involved in
initiative, control, responsibillity, and combat, would
have been enough in itself to have absorbed the
whole efforts of at least two lives of ordinary vigour.
And at the same time her work in connection with
India, which had begun with the Sanitary
Commission on the Indian Army, spread and
ramified in a multitude of directions. Her tentacles
reached the India Office and succeeded in
establishing a hold even upon those slippery high
places. For many years it was de rigueur for the
newly appointed Viceroy, before he left England, to
pay a visit to Miss Nightingale.

After much hesitation, she had settled down in a small house in South Street, where she remained for the rest of her life. That life was a very long one; the dying woman reached her ninety- first year. Her ill health gradually diminished; the crises of extreme danger became less frequent, and at last altogether ceased; she remained an invalid, but an invalid of a curious character—an invalid who was too weak to walk downstairs and who worked far harder than most Cabinet Ministers. Her illness, whatever it may have been, was certainly not inconvenient. It involved seclusion; and an extraordinary, an unparalleled seclusion was, it might almost have been said, the mainspring of Miss Nightingale's life. Lying on her sofa in the little upper room in South Street, she combined the intense vitality of a dominating woman of the world with the mysterious and romantic quality of a myth. She was a legend in her lifetime, and she knew it. She tasted the joys of power, like those Eastern Emperors whose autocratic rule was based upon invisibility, with the mingled satisfactions of obscurity and fame.

And she found the machinery of illness hardly less effective as a barrier against the eyes of men than the ceremonial of a palace. Great statesmen and renowned generals were obliged to beg for audiences; admiring princesses from foreign countries found that they must see her at her own time, or not at all; and the ordinary mortal had no hope of ever getting beyond the downstairs sitting-room and Dr. Sutherland. For that indefatigable disciple did, indeed, never desert her. He might be impatient, he might be restless, but he remained. His 'incurable looseness of thought', for so she termed it, continued at her service to the end. Once, it is true, he had actually ventured to take a holiday; but he was recalled, and he did not repeat the experiment. He was wanted downstairs. There he sat, transacting business answering correspondence, interviewing callers, and exchanging innumerable notes with the unseen power above. Sometimes word came down that Miss Nightingale was just well enough to see one of her visitors. The fortunate man was led up, was ushered, trembling, into the shaded chamber, and, of course, could never afterwards forget the interview. Very rarely, indeed, once or twice a year, perhaps, but nobody could be quite certain, in deadly secrecy, Miss Nightingale went out for a drive in the Park. Unrecognised, the living legend flitted for a moment before the common gaze. And the precaution was necessary; for there were times when, at some public function, the rumour of her presence was spread abroad; and ladies, mistaken by the crowd for Miss Nightingale, were followed, pressed upon, vehemently supplicated 'Let me touch your shawl'; 'Let me stroke your arm'; such was the strange adoration in the hearts of the people. That vast reserve of force lay there behind her; she could use it, if she could. But she preferred never to use it. On occasions, she might hint or threaten, she might balance the sword of Damocles over the head of the Bison; she might, by a word, by a glance, remind some refractory Minister, some unpersuadable Viceroy, sitting in audience with her in the little upper room, that she was something more than a mere sick woman, that she had only, so to speak, to go to the window and wave her handkerchief, for ... dreadful things to follow. But that was enough; they understood; the myth was there- -obvious, portentous, impalpable; and so it remained to the last.

With statesmen and governors at her beck and call, with her hands on a hundred strings, with mighty provinces at her feet, with foreign governments agog for her counsel, building hospitals, training nurses— she still felt that she had not enough to do. She sighed for more worlds to conquer—more, and yet more.

She looked about her—what was left? Of course! Philosophy! After the world of action, the world of thought. Having set right the health of the British Army, she would now do the same good service for the religious convictions of mankind. She had long noticed—with regret—the growing tendency towards free-thinking among artisans. With regret, but not altogether with surprise, the current teaching of Christianity was sadly to seek; nay, Christianity itself was not without its defects. She would rectify these errors. She would correct the mistakes of the Churches; she would point out just where Christianity was wrong; and she would explain to the artisans what the facts of the case really were. Before her departure for the Crimea, she had begun this work; and now, in the intervals of her other labours, she completed it. Her 'Suggestions for Thought to the Searchers After

Truth Among the Artisans of England' (1860), unravels, in the course of three portly volumes, the difficulties hitherto, curiously enough, unsolved—connected with such matters as Belief in God, the Plan of Creation, the Origin of Evil, the Future Life, Necessity and Free Will, Law, and the Nature of Morality.

The Origin of Evil, in particular, held no perplexities for Miss Nightingale. 'We cannot conceive,' she remarks, 'that Omnipotent Righteousness would find satisfaction in solitary existence.' This being, so, the only question remaining to be asked is: 'What beings should we then conceive that God would create?' Now, He cannot create perfect beings, 'since, essentially, perfection is one'; if He did so, He would only be adding to Himself. Thus the conclusion is obvious: He must create imperfect ones. Omnipotent Righteousness, faced by the intolerable impasse of a solitary existence, finds itself bound by the very nature of the cause, to create the hospitals at Scutari. Whether this argument would have satisfied the artisans was never discovered, for only a very few copies of the book were printed for private circulation. One copy was sent to Mr. Mill, who acknowledged it in an extremely polite letter. He felt himself obliged, however, to confess that he had not been altogether convinced by Miss Nightingale's proof of the existence of God. Miss Nightingale was surprised and mortified; she had thought better of Mr. Mill; for surely her proof of the existence of God could hardly be improved upon. 'A law,' she had pointed out, 'implies a lawgiver.' Now the Universe is full of laws—the law of gravitation, the law of the excluded middle, and many others; hence it follows that the Universe has a law-giver— and what would Mr. Mill be satisfied with, if he was not satisfied with that?

Perhaps Mr. Mill might have asked why the argument had not been pushed to its logical conclusion. Clearly, if we are to trust the analogy of human institutions, we must remember that laws are, as a matter of fact, not dispensed by lawgivers, but passed by Act of Parliament. Miss Nightingale, however, with all her experience of public life, never stopped to consider the question whether God might not be a Limited Monarchy.Yet her conception of

God was certainly not orthodox. She felt towards Him as she might have felt towards a glorified sanitary engineer; and in some of her speculations she seems hardly to distinguish between the Deity and the Drains. As one turns over these singular pages, one has the impression that Miss Nightingale has got the Almighty too into her clutches, and that, if He is not careful, she will kill Him with overwork.

Then, suddenly, in the very midst of the ramifying generalities of her metaphysical disquisitions, there is an unexpected turn and the reader is plunged all at once into something particular, something personal, something impregnated with intense experience— a virulent invective upon the position of women in the upper ranks of society. Forgetful alike of her high argument and of the artisans, the bitter creature rails through a hundred pages of close print at the falsities of family life, the ineptitudes of marriage, the emptinesses of convention, in the spirit of an Ibsen or a Samuel Butler. Her fierce pen, shaking with intimate anger, depicts in biting sentences the fearful fate of an unmarried girl in a wealthy household. It is a cri du coeur; and then, as suddenly, she returns once more to instruct the artisans upon the nature ofOmnipotent Righteousness.

Her mind was, indeed, better qualified to dissect the concrete and distasteful fruits of actual life than to construct a coherent system of abstract philosophy. In spite of her respect for Law, she was never at home with a generalisation. Thus, though the great achievement of her life lay in the immense impetus which she gave to the scientific treatment of sickness, a true comprehension of the scientific method itself was alien to her spirit. Like most great men of action—perhaps like all—she was simply an empiricist. She believed in what she saw, and she acted accordingly; beyond that she would not go. She had found in Scutari that fresh air and light played an effective part in the prevention of the maladies with which she had to deal; and that was enough for her; she would not inquire further; what were the general principles underlying that fact—or even whether there were any—she refused to consider. Years after the discoveries of Pasteur and Lister, she laughed at what she called the 'germ- fetish'. There was no such thing as 'infection'; she had never seen it, therefore it did not exist. But she had seen the good effects of fresh air; therefore, there could be no doubt about them; and therefore, it was essential that the bedrooms of patients should be well ventilated. Such was her doctrine; and in those days of hermetically scaled windows it was a very valuable one. But it was a purely empirical doctrine, and thus it led to some unfortunate results. When, for instance, her influence in India was at its height, she issued orders that all hospital windows should be invariably kept open. The authorities, who knew what an open window in the hot weather meant, protested, but in vain; Miss Nightingale was incredulous. She knew nothing of the hot weather, but she did know the value of fresh air—from personal experience; the authorities were talking nonsense; and the windows must be kept open all the year round. There was a great outcry from all the doctors in India, but she was firm; and for a moment it seemed possible that her terrible commands would have to be put into execution. Lord Lawrence, however, was Viceroy, and he was able to intimate to Miss Nightingale, with sufficient authority, that himself had decided upon the question, and that his decision must stand, even against her own. Upon that she gave way, but reluctantly and quite unconvinced; she was only puzzled by the unexpected weakness of Lord Lawrence. No doubt, if she had lived today, and if her experience had lain, not among cholera cases at Scutari, but among yellow-fever cases in Panama, she would have declared fresh air a fetish, and would have maintained to her dying day that the only really effective way of dealing with disease was by the destruction of mosquitoes.

Yet her mind, so positive, so realistic, so ultra-practical, had its singular revulsions, its mysterious moods of mysticism and of doubt. At times, lying sleepless in the early hours, she fell into long, strange, agonised meditations, and then, seizing a pencil, she would commit to paper the confessions of her soul. The morbid longings of her pre-Crimean days came over her once more; she filled page after page with self-examination, self-criticism, self-surrender. 'Oh Father,' she wrote, 'I submit, I resign myself, I accept with all my heart, thisstretching out of Thy hand to save me. ... Oh how vain it is, the vanity of vanities, to live in men's thoughts instead of God's!'

She was lonely, she was miserable. 'Thou knowest that through all these horrible twenty years, I have been supported by the belief that I was working with Thee who would bring everyone, even our poor nurses, to perfection'—and yet, after all, what was the result? Had not even she been an unprofitable servant? One night, waking suddenly, she saw, in the dim light of the night-lamp, tenebrous shapes upon the wall. The past rushed back upon her. 'Am I she who once stood on that Crimean height?' she wildly asked— "The Lady with a lamp shall stand . . .The lamp shows me only my utter shipwreck.'

She sought consolation in the writings of the Mystics and in a correspondence with Mr. Jowett. For many years the Master of Balliol acted as her spiritual adviser. He discussed with her in a series of enormous letters the problems of religion and philosophy; he criticised her writings on those subjects with the tactful sympathy of a cleric who was also a man of the world; and he even ventured to attempt at times to instil into her rebellious nature some of his own peculiar suavity. 'I sometimes think,' he told her, 'that you ought seriously to consider how your work may be carried on, not with less energy, but in a calmer spirit. I am not blaming the past... But I want the peace of God to settle on the future.' He recommended her to spend her time no longer in 'conflicts with Government offices', and to take up some literary work. He urged her to 'work out her notion of Divine Perfection', in a series of essays for Frazer's Magazine. She did so; and the result was submitted to Mr. Froude, who pronounced the second essay to be 'even more pregnant than the first. I cannot tell,' he said, 'how sanitary, with disordered intellects, the effects of such papers will be.'

Mr. Carlyle, indeed, used different language, and some remarks of his about a lost lamb bleating on the mountains, having been unfortunately repeated to Miss Nightingale, required all Mr. Jowett's suavity to keep the peace. In a letter of fourteen sheets, he turned her attention from this painful topic towards a discussion of Quietism. 'I don't see why,' said the Master of Balliol, 'active life might not become a sort of passive life too.' And then, he added, 'I sometimes fancy there are possibilities of human character much greater than have been realised.' She found such sentiments helpful, underlining them in blue pencil; and, in return, she assisted her friend with a long series of elaborate comments upon the Dialogues of Plato, most of which he embodied in the second edition of his translation. Gradually her interest became more personal; she told him never to work again after midnight, and he obeyed her. Then she helped him to draw up a special form of daily service for the College Chapel, with selections from the Psalms under the heads of 'God the Lord, God the judge, God the Father, and God the Friend'— though, indeed, this project was never realised; for the Bishop of Oxford disallowed the alterations, exercising his legal powers, on the advice of Sir Travers Twiss.

Their relations became intimate. 'The spirit of the Twenty-third Psalm and the spirit of the Nineteenth Psalm should be united in our lives,' Mr. Jowett said. Eventually, she asked him to do her a singular favour. Would he, knowing what he did of her religious views, come to London and administer to her the Holy Sacrament? He did not hesitate, and afterwards declared that he would always regard the occasion as a solemn event in his life. He was devoted to her— though the precise nature of his feelings towards her never quite transpired. Her feelings towards him were more mixed. At first, he was 'that great and good man'—'that true saint, Mr. Jowett'; but, as time went on, some gall was mingled with the balm; the acrimony of her nature asserted itself. She felt that she gave more sympathy than she received; she was exhausted, and she was annoyed by his conversation. Her tongue, one day, could not refrain from shooting out at him: 'He comes to me, and he talks to me,' she said, 'as if I were someone else.'

V

AT one time she had almost decided to end her life in retirement as a patient at St. Thomas's Hospital. But partly owing to the persuasions of Mr. Jowett, she changed her mind; for forty-five years she remained in South Street; and in South Street she died. As old age approached, though her influence with the official world gradually diminished, her activities seemed to remain as intense and widespread as before. When hospitals were to be built, when schemes of sanitary reform were in agitation, when wars broke out, she was still the adviser of all Europe. Still, with a characteristic self-assurance, she watched from her Mayfair bedroom over the welfare of India. Still, with an indefatigable enthusiasm, she pushed forward the work, which, perhaps, was nearer to her heart, more completely her own, than all the rest— the training of nurses. In her moments of deepest depression, when her greatest achievements seemed to lose their lustre, she thought of her nurses, and was comforted. The ways of God, she found, were strange indeed. 'How inefficient I was in the Crimea,' she noted. 'Yet He has raised up from it trained nursing.'

At other times, she was better satisfied. Looking back, she was amazed by the enormous change which, since her early days, had come over the whole treatment of illness, the whole conception of public and domestic health—a change in which, she knew, she had played her part. One of her Indian admirers, the Aga Khan, came to visit her. She expatiated on the marvellous advances she had lived to see in the management of hospitals— in drainage, in ventilation, in sanitary work of every kind. There was a pause; and then, 'Do you think you are improving?' asked the Aga Khan. She was a little taken aback, and said, 'What do you mean by "improving"?' He replied, 'Believing more in God.' She saw that he had a view of God which was different from hers. 'A most interesting man,' she noted after the interview; 'but you could never teach him sanitation.'

When old age actually came, something curious happened. Destiny, having waited very patiently, played a queer trick on Miss Nightingale. The benevolence and public spirit of that long life had only been equalled by its acerbity. Her virtue had dwelt in hardness, and she had poured forth her unstinted usefulness with a bitter smile upon her lips. And now the sarcastic years brought the proud woman her punishment. She was not to die as she had lived. The sting was to be taken out of her; she was to be made soft; she was to be reduced to compliance and complacency. The change came gradually, but at last it was unmistakable. The terrible commander who had driven Sidney Herbert to his death, to whom Mr. Jowett had applied the words of Homer, amoton memaniia— raging insatiably— now accepted small compliments with gratitude, and indulged in sentimental friendships with young girls. The author of "Notes on Nursing"—that classical compendium of the besetting sins of the sisterhood, drawn up with the detailed acrimony, the vindictive relish, of a Swift—now spent long hours in composing sympathetic Addresses to Probationers, whom she petted and wept over in turn. And, at the same time, there appeared a corresponding alteration in her physical mood. The thin, angular woman, with her haughty eye and her acrid mouth, had vanished; and in her place was the rounded, bulky form of a fat old lady, smiling all day long. Then something else became visible. The brain which had been steeled at Scutari was indeed, literally, growing soft. Senility—an ever more and more amiable senility—descended. Towards the end, consciousness itself grew lost in a roseate haze, and melted into nothingness.

It was just then, three years before her death, when she was eighty-seven years old (1907), that those in authority bethought them that the opportune moment had come for bestowing a public honour on Florence Nightingale. She was offered the Order of Merit. That Order, whose roll contains, among other distinguished names, those of Sir Lawrence Alma Tadema and Sir Edward Elgar, is remarkable chiefly for the fact that, as its title indicates, it is bestowed because its recipient deserves it, and for no other reason. Miss Nightingale's representatives accepted the honour, and her name, after a lapse of many years, once more appeared in the Press. Congratulations from all sides came pouring in. There was a universal burst of enthusiasm—a final revivification of the ancient myth. Among her other admirers, the German Emperor took this opportunity of expressing his feelings towards her. 'His Majesty,' wrote the German Ambassador, 'having just brought to a close a most enjoyable stay in the beautiful neighbourhood of your old home near Romsey, has commanded me to present you with some flowers as a token of his esteem.' Then, by Royal command, the Order of Merit was brought to South Street, and there was a little ceremony of presentation. Sir Douglas Dawson, after a short speech, stepped forward, and handed the insignia of the Order to Miss Nightingale. Propped up by pillows, she dimly recognised that some compliment was being paid

her. 'Too kind— too kind,' she murmured; and she
was not ironical.

BIBLIOGRAPHY
Sir E. Cook. Life of Florence Nightingale.
A. W. Kinglake. The Invasion of the Crimea.
Lord Sidney Godolphin Osborne. Scutari and its
Hospitals.
S. M. Mitra. Life of Sir John Hall.
Lord Stanmore. Sidney Herbert.
Sir G. Douglas. The Panmure Papers.
Sir H. Maxwell. Life and Letters of the Fourth
Earl of Clarendon.
E.Abbott and L. Campbell. Life and Letters of
Benjamin Jowett.   A.H.   Clough. Poems and
Memoir.

Made in the USA